THE BASIC MENTAL HEALTH GOALS

Daily Habits to Build and Strengthen your Mental Toughness

NORAU.I

Contents

INTRODUCTION

Our emotional, psychological, and social well-being are all parts of our mental health. It influences our thoughts, emotions, and behaviors. Additionally, it influences how we respond to stress, interact with others, and make good decisions. Every period of life, from childhood and adolescence to maturity, is vital for mental health.

Poor mental health and mental illness are not the same things, despite the fact that the phrases are sometimes used synonymously. Even if they may not have a mental disorder, a person can have poor mental health. A person with a mental illness may also go through periods of good physical, mental, and social health.

Why is mental health crucial to general well-being?

Both physical and mental health are crucial aspects of overall health. For instance, depression raises the danger of many different physical health issues, especially chronic diseases like diabetes, heart disease, and stroke. In a similar vein, having chronic illnesses raises your likelihood of developing mental disease.

Can the state of your mind change over time?

It is crucial to keep in mind that a person's mental health can alter over time and depend on a variety of circumstances. A person's mental health may be affected if the demands placed on them are greater than their capacity for coping and resources. For instance, someone may have poor mental health if they are working long hours, providing care for a relative, or going through financial difficulties.

How widespread are mental disorders?

One of the most prevalent medical problems in the US is mental illness.

At some point in their lives, more than 50% of people will receive a diagnosis of a mental illness or disorder.

In any given year, 1 in 5 Americans will suffer from a mental illness.

A severely disabling mental illness affects 1 in 5 children either now or at some point in their lives.

A significant mental illness like schizophrenia, bipolar disorder, or major depression affects 1 in 25 people in the United States.

Why does mental disease occur?

Mental illness has many causes, not just one. The likelihood of mental disease can be influenced by a variety of circumstances, including

Early traumatic events in life or a history of maltreatment (for example, child abuse, sexual assault, witnessing violence, etc.)

Experiences with other persistent (chronic) illnesses, such cancer or diabetes

Biological components or brain chemical imbalances

Use of drugs or alcohol

Experiencing emotions of isolation or loneliness

CHAPTER 1

Ideas about mental health

Mental health is a condition of mental wellness that enables people to manage life's stressors, develop their potential, study and work effectively, and give back to their communities. It is a crucial element of health and well-being that supports both our individual and group capacity to decide, form connections, and influence the world we live in. A core human right is access to mental health. Additionally, it is essential for socioeconomic, communal, and personal development.

The absence of mental diseases is only one aspect of mental wellness. It has variable degrees of difficulty and suffering, is experienced differently by each individual, and may have very different social and therapeutic implications. It exists on a complex continuum.

Mental health issues include psychosocial impairments, mental illnesses, and other mental states linked to high levels of suffering, functional limitations, or risk of self-harm. Although this is not always or necessarily the case, people with mental health disorders are more likely to have lower levels of mental well-being.

Factors that affect mental health

Numerous individual, social, and structural factors may interact throughout our lives to support or undermine our mental health and cause a change in where we fall on the mental health continuum.

People may be more susceptible to mental health issues due to personal psychological and biological characteristics like emotional intelligence, substance use, and heredity.

People are more likely to develop mental health issues when they are exposed to unfavorable social, economic, geopolitical, and environmental conditions, such as poverty, violence, inequality, and environmental squalor.

Risks can appear at any stage of life, but those that happen during developmentally vulnerable times, notably early childhood, are most harmful. For instance, physical punishment and strict parenting are known to harm children's health, and bullying is a major risk factor for mental health issues.

Similar protective factors persist throughout our lives and help us be more resilient. They comprise, among other things, our unique social and emotional capacities and characteristics as well as satisfying interpersonal relationships, high-quality education, respectable employment, secure neighborhoods, and cohesive communities.

At various scales, society contains both threats and safeguards for mental health. Risk for individuals, families, and communities is increased by local threats. Global risks, which include economic downturns, disease outbreaks, humanitarian crises, forced displacement, and the escalating climate issue, raise the risk for entire populations.

Only a few risk and protective factors can be reliably predicted. Despite being exposed to a risk factor, the majority of people do not go on to acquire a mental health illness, while many people who have no known risk factor do so nonetheless. However, the interrelated factors that affect mental health can either support or detract from it.

Prevention and promotion of mental illness

In order to lower risks, foster resilience, and create environments that are supportive of mental health, promotion and prevention interventions first identify the individual, societal, and structural determinants of mental health. Interventions may be created for single people, particular groups, or entire populations.

Promotion and prevention programs should encompass the education, labor, justice, transportation, environment, housing, and welfare sectors since changing the determinants of mental health frequently requires action beyond the health sector. By integrating promotion and preventive initiatives into health services, as well as by advocating, starting, and, when necessary, supporting multispectral collaboration and coordination, the health sector may make a substantial contribution.

Globally important and covered under the Sustainable Development Goals is the prevention of suicide. Limiting access to resources, responsible media coverage, social and emotional learning for teenagers, and early intervention can all result in significant progress. A very low-cost and cost-effective technique for lowering suicide rates is banning highly dangerous chemicals.

Another objective is to support caregivers in providing nurturing care. This can be done by enacting laws and policies that support and safeguard mental health, developing school-based programs, and enhancing community and online environments. Programs for social and emotional development that are taught in schools are among the best ways for nations of all income levels to advance their economies.

Growing interest in the promotion and protection of mental health at work can be supported by laws and regulations, organizational tactics, manager training, and worker interventions.

CHAPTER TWO

Logical goals for mental health

Setting SMART objectives requires consciously acknowledging and identifying your goals as well as developing a methodical plan to make achieving them easier. This book will demonstrate how to use Mooditude's Goals & Routines habit-building tool to make manageable mental health goals.

We are constantly occupied with work, school, and household duties. We have a routine that we adhere to, and for the most part, we believe that we are aware of what we are doing, why we are doing it, and what we hope to accomplish. There are, however, times of relief when you may finally pause from life and unwind. You prepare a beautiful cup of coffee, put some relaxing music on in the background, decide to reward yourself, and then sit on the sofa and watch your favorite movie when suddenly, reality hits you like a ton of bricks.

Setting goals is the process by which the aforementioned person or group plans to accomplish the desired goal. Goal setting entails a conscious acknowledgment and identification of your goals and a meticulous strategy to make it easier to achieve these goals by taking control of life instead of living passively. This contrasts with having a vague idea of what your desired goal is and living life passively, hoping to achieve it someway without a proper plan.

Setting Mental Health Objectives

Setting personal goals for treatment is a fantastic method to get past some mental health obstacles because the main goal of goal setting is to stimulate growth and success in the recovery and mental healthcare professions. Lack of energy, motivation, a general reduction in performance, and a loss of interest in activities are all symptoms of poor mental health. It's a wonderful idea to set goals and create plans and methods to achieve them in order to regain lost motivation and gradually enhance overall mental health.

Setting personal objectives and working toward them can also help persons with poor mental health recover control over their lives because they might feel like they have lost it. Various psychotherapies, including Cognitive-Behavioral Therapy (CBT), Interpersonal Psychotherapy, Problem-Solving Therapy, etc., frequently employ goal-setting as a component.

Different Goals

Goal setting is a tried-and-true technique in the field of mental healthcare for monitoring patient progress and promoting healing by assisting patients in defining and achieving realistic goals. Goals can, in general, be classified as long-term or short-term.

Short-term Objectives

Short-term objectives typically address immediate needs, are simpler to accomplish, and don't take much work. Short-term objectives are frequently aimed to help you get closer to your ultimate goal or long-term purpose. They serve as a constant source of inspiration and reduce the difficulty of accomplishing long-term or ultimate goals. They aid in retaining attention,

Monitoring performance, and identifying areas that require improvement. For instance, if your goal is to read ten novels in two months, you'll inevitably find the work overwhelming and more prone to procrastination. In contrast, setting a goal to read two chapters of a single book every day may not seem like a difficult one at all, and you may even manage to go beyond it.

Long-Term Objectives

Long-term goals are less precise and have a greater scope than short-term goals. Typically, you want to accomplish these chores in the future. These goals call both meticulous planning and ongoing motivation, both of which can be attained through achieving short-term objectives. Long-term objectives provide direction for your life and let you plan ahead. For instance, a long-term objective can be to strengthen your bonds with friends or family. This takes a lot of effort, time, and patience and cannot be completed quickly.

Five Advantages of Goal-Setting

Setting goals is essential for encouraging personal development. Setting goals has many advantages, regardless of whether they are intended to be a kind of treatment for mental health issues or merely methods to enhance your quality of life.

1. Provides guidance

Setting objectives gives one direction. It gives you a target to shoot your fictitious arrow at so you aren't passively and aimlessly meandering through life. Once the direction is known, planning a path or a strategy to get there is simpler.

2. Constant Source of Motivation

Setting objectives, particularly short-term ones, might help you stay motivated. When dealing with a mental health problem, it's typically simple to lose motivation, direction, and concentration. Regularly working toward achieving short-term goals ensures a steady source of motivation.

3. Offers a Sharp focus

When faced with difficulties, it is simple to become distracted in life. People who have mental health problems frequently lose sight of their goals in life and become mired in unendingly depressing thoughts about them. Setting goals can aid in removing the depression's haze and enabling you to concentrate clearly on your main aim.

4. Provides life control

Many persons with mental health issues seem to believe that their mental illness has taken control of their lives and that they no longer have any control over it. One might feel more in control of their life by setting attainable goals.

5. Encourages Confidence

Low self-esteem and confidence in oneself are common among people with depression and anxiety. They can gain the confidence boost they sorely need when they are able to achieve something on their own.

Setting Realistic Objectives

Setting objectives is a difficult endeavor, but it becomes simpler when you divide it into manageable chunks. You start by figuring out the overall picture, or the ultimate goal you want to achieve by the end of a certain amount of time, and then you break it down into smaller, more manageable pieces. Following are some recommendations on how to develop achievable objectives that can enhance your mental well-being.

The SMART Method

The SMART approach makes sure that each goals you set for yourself is well thought out and measurable. The acronym SMART stands for:

S = Precise: Your goals should be small and specific rather than broad so that you may more easily strategize how to attain it by creating a strategy that is tailored to the particular aim.

I'll repair my relationship with my parents, for instance.

M= Setting quantifiable, or easily traceable, goals is a crucial component of creating realistic goals. You can determine whether your method is effective by setting checkpoints to gauge your progress.

For instance, I'll try to see my parents at least three times a week as I work to repair our relationship.

A = Achievable: Objectives ought to always be reachable. Being too hard on yourself can make you fail because you are the best person to know your potential. Self-awareness is very important for this. It also implies that you are completely aware of and prepared to take the necessary steps to accomplish that goal.

For instance, I'll aim to see my parents at least three times per week while resolving the challenges brought on by my anger issues.

R = Relevant: When setting a goal, it's important that it be related to your overall life objective and, as a result, should help you get there in the long term.

Example: In order to reach my objective of resolving my behavioral difficulties, I will endeavor to resolve the challenges brought on by my anger issues and make an effort to see my parents at least three times per week.

T = Time-Based: It's important to set a deadline for achieving your desired result. An end-date serves as a continuous source of inspiration and helps you stay on task.

By addressing the challenges brought on by my anger issues and making an effort to see my parents at least three times each week, for instance, I will start the process of resolving my behavioral issues by mending my relationship with my parents within a month.

How Does Mooditude's Goal-Setting Process Work?

A mental health resource called Mooditude helps you find happiness in a secure environment. It offers resources for creating goals, self-care, mood monitoring, and mental health screening. You may establish and track short-term objectives with Mooditude's variety of challenges and activities to stay motivated.

You can choose from a variety of tasks on Mooditude, and you can keep track of your progress as you go. It also provides guidance on how frequently a task should be performed to enhance mental health on a specific day, according to professional recommendations. Mooditude offers a number of objectives, including:

1. Journaling

You can challenge yourself to write in your journal 1–5 times every day. A tried-and-true method for coping with mental health problems is journaling. For greatest results, Mooditude suggests keeping a journal at least once every day.

2. Meditation

Mooditude advises maintaining a schedule to meditate and develop mindfulness. Just 10 minutes of daily meditation, broken up into periods of 3 minutes, 2 minutes, and 5 minutes each in the morning, afternoon, and evening, can provide noticeable results.

If you want to work on your objectives for extended periods of time, you can define your own targets.

3. Exercise

It's essential to stay physically active to keep your mind healthy. However, maintaining a schedule might be challenging. Fortunately, a noticeable increase in mental health can be shown after just 10 minutes of action, such as brisk walking. To prevent slacking off, make it a point to exercise for at least 10 minutes each day.

4. Sleep

Sleep habits can be significantly impacted by mental health, leaving you groggy all day. The link between depression and sleeplessness has been demonstrated by research. The Centers for Disease Control and Prevention (CDC) estimate that a healthy night's sleep for an adult is between 7-8 hours. Establish a goal for getting enough sleep, and monitor how frequently you wake up during the night.

5. Exercises for Cognitive Behavioral Therapy (CBT):

By assisting with coping with and challenging irrational negative beliefs through a number of straightforward exercises, CBT exercises can help combat a variety of mental health conditions, including depression, anxiety, and low self-esteem. One CBT exercise each day, according to Mooditude, is an acceptable objective.

6. Mindfulness

In addition to enhancing relationships, living a mindful life can also boost emotions of wellbeing, lessen emotional reactivity, heighten empathy, and enhance emotional processing abilities. Activities that promote mindfulness are easy and enjoyable. For novices, it is appropriate to establish a goal of being attentive at least twice or three times every day.

7. Social Networking

Isolation can be detrimental, and mental diseases can be isolating. In order to preserve social relationships, Mooditude advises choosing a goal that is simple to achieve: communicate with loved ones, friends, acquaintances, or total strangers.

8. Gratitude

Gratitude exercises can increase levels of activity while reducing stress and anxiety. Being thankful helps you to let go of the past and live in the moment rather than being mired in regret. The daily practice of counting your blessings should be one of your goals.

9. Limit caffeine consumption

No matter how prevalent coffee drinking may be, it has been shown to be associated with greater levels of stress, anxiety, and depression. One cup of coffee can worsen anxiety and have a 48-hour negative effect on sleep. Mooditude can assist in defining a personal goal to reduce coffee consumption and tracking progress, even though it may be a difficult task to complete.

10. Obtain sunlight

A fantastic therapeutic option for SAD, anxiety, despair, and other conditions is light therapy. It can help with mood enhancement, reviving energy, and addressing sleep issues. While our indoor time may be limited by busy schedules, having a goal can inspire us to get outside and enjoy the sunshine.

11. Medicine

When taken over an extended period of time, medications can change the brain's neurotransmitters that control mood. Setting goals can help persons with mood and anxiety disorders brought on by medication stay on track and identify the medicine that is to blame for their condition.

12. Limit Abuse of Substances

We must engage in activities that are good for our bodies as well as our brains in order for the brain to heal. We must also reduce the detrimental behaviors and practices we engage in. One of the main causes of many mental health problems is substance addiction. Setting a personal limit on substance usage can help reduce it all the way to zero over time.

Reevaluating and Reevaluating Goals

It is useless to just create goals at the beginning of the year and never go back to evaluate, reassess, or monitor your progress toward them. Reviewing your objectives can assist in determining whether they are still important, whether your plan has proven successful, and whether you have made any progress. It can also help you decide if you're prepared to go past easy objectives and set more difficult ones that could demand more work.

Depending on the type of objective you have established, you should evaluate it more frequently. Regardless, it should be understood that frequent visits are the best course of action. Checking in every 5-7 days is advised for short-term goals that act as stepping stones towards the long-term objective.

CHAPTER THREE

Daily routine for battling depression

Many people have found it tough to get out of bed or find the motivation to start the day because of depression. A good daily regimen, though, can make life a whole lot simpler. Following and putting into practice your daily routines might assist you in escaping, even when you feel as though you are being drawn into a gloomy void.

Everyday tasks become more difficult when you have depression, and the symptoms make you feel unloved, unworthy, and alone.

Are you aware that about 5% of Americans experience depression? Therefore, keep in mind that you're not alone despite how much sadness makes you feel lonely.

Treatment and recovery from depression are feasible with professional assistance, therapy, medication, or a mix of talk therapy and medication. What can you do, though, to prevent your depressive symptoms while these treatments are working?

Ah, the routine! Maintaining a regular, healthy routine can assist you in overcoming depression. Here are the top 10 daily regular activities for battling and preventing depression.

Depression Daily Routine: Things You Must Try

1. Your alarm clock is a close friend.

Clock-Is-Your-Best-Buddy

It's vital to keep in mind the link between sleep and mental wellness. Lack of sleep has been associated with a higher chance of developing depression. Even if your sleep schedule is inconsistent, it can raise your risk of developing depression. The quality as well as the amount of sleep we get, therefore make your alarm clock your closest buddy!

Try to maintain a consistent sleep and waking schedule each day. You can combat the signs of depression by maintaining a regular sleep routine. Decide on a time and set an alarm. You lose if you sleep, after all.

2. Your Diet Is Important!

Once more, how you eat affects how you manage your depression. Are you aware that eating processed meals can make depression more likely? It's okay to consume them in moderation, but it's not ideal to incorporate an unhealthy diet into your daily routine. You must record your food intake.

Add some protein to your lunch, some fresh fruit to your breakfast, and some vegetables to your dinner. Supplements including zinc and vitamin D may also be added to your regular regimen in order to lessen the symptoms of depression.

*Please remember that you should consult a doctor to discuss any possible risks and side effects before taking supplements. Additional supplements taken in excess can be dangerous.

3. Move! Move! Move! Never stop moving; continue on.

Well, it can be difficult to persuade oneself to move when you're dealing with despair. Nevertheless, adding it to a sad person's daily routine is a terrific idea. Exercises like yoga, running, and cardio can help boost endorphin production and lessen depressive symptoms. Additionally, you can exercise without a membership to a gym. Every day, go for a 10-minute jog while wearing your running shoes. You can up your workout to moderate intensity when you're ready, for at least one hour. Adding hobbies to your daily routine to help with depression includes things like gardening, playing with your pets, and dancing for no one.

4. Quite literally, water is life.

Drinking water and staying hydrated are two tasks that are easy to add to your daily schedule. Even though it may not appear to be the case, drinking water throughout the day can help to lessen the signs and symptoms of depression.

You can carry a water bottle or set up a phone notification to remind you to stay hydrated as part of this daily practice.

5. Develop a Journaling Habit

The barrage of unfavorable ideas and beliefs is a significant contributor to depression that we experience. You can communicate such emotions and thoughts through journaling. Did you realize that simply making a list might be beneficial? For this habit, you don't have to keep a journal. This daily habit seems to work fairly well to me because you can select when, where, and how to journal.

Simply include journaling in your daily routine for at least five minutes each day, preferably before bed or in the morning. Here are a few brief starters to get you going:

Give your loved ones a list of three things you wish to say.

List the toughest feelings you frequently go through.

Describe three things that make you happy.

6. Shut your eyes and begin to relax

It is challenging to just be and slow down. It can be challenging to stop overanalyzing and feeling overwhelmed, but it is necessary for your mental health. Make it a habit to incorporate meditation into your everyday routine in between therapy sessions. You only need to sit quietly, close your eyes, and simply...be.

You can choose a time when you're the least distracted and only concentrate on your breathing to include this exercise into your everyday schedule. You can meditate to decompress at the end of the day or to start your day off well in the morning.

7. Remember To Say "Thank You"

Particularly if you're depressed, it can be simpler to concentrate on the negatives than the advantages. Negative ideas are quite prevalent, but you can't always allow them rule your mind. So let's incorporate feeling grateful for surviving depression into our everyday routine to lessen their intensity.

All you have to do is express gratitude for the tiny things in life. Saying "Thank you" to the universe, the barista from whom you get your daily coffee, a flower that made you smile, or just to yourself might be included in this. Take some time each day to express your gratitude because we all have things and people for whom we are thankful.

8. After All, Kindness Is a Virtue

Taking care of others' needs and wants may be the last thing on a person's mind when they are depressed, but did you know that doing so can hasten your recovery? Don't just concentrate on yourself; spread your generosity as well!

Additionally, it will make you happy to know that your kind deed made someone else's day. Saying thank you, holding doors for others, or purchasing a cup of coffee for someone can all be small acts of kindness that can uplift and cheer you. Being kind is always worthwhile.

9. The best care is self-care

Self-care is a straightforward yet extremely powerful action that a depressed person should add to their daily routine. Self-care practices like deep breathing exercises, meditation, and even a warm bath can help lessen the effects of depression.

Simple techniques like massage therapy, music therapy, or aromatherapy can be included into your regular routine. You might also include routines like:

Reading a section of your preferred book

After a long day, taking a hot bath

Taking care of one's physique and skin

Playing with your animal friend

Any activity that promotes relaxation at the end of the day is fine. The only guideline for self-care is to unwind and have fun.

10. Finally, relax and take it easy.

Depression is an illness that can strike without warning and can completely disrupt your daily schedule. You must constantly remind yourself that depression manifests in unpredictable ways, just like other medical illnesses. As with any physical ailment, depression symptoms should be handled with care and consideration.

Take it easy, and don't be too hard on yourself if you can't keep up with your depression-fighting daily regimen. Try to relax on your terms and give yourself some time. Keep in mind that you can always get counseling and expert support. Put your attention on relaxing and taking care of yourself. That is what fuels us.

CHAPTER FOUR

How to increase mental toughness

We constantly put our mental fortitude to the test. You can be struggling with a loved one's death or losing your job.

Additionally, mental health is distinct from mental toughness or resilience.

Some people might assume that when they hear the terms "mental strength" or "resiliency," it means they do not have a mental disease, but this is not the case. Many people who suffer from mental illness have developed appropriate coping mechanisms. They have developed emotional resilience and enjoy good mental health. Similar to this, a person can have both poor mental health and low emotional resilience without ever having experienced mental illness.

What is a mental toughness?

How well someone handles difficulties, demands, and stressors they may experience is a measure of their mental strength or emotional resilience.

Enhancing your mental fortitude can improve life satisfaction and ward off future mental health problems.

Why is that crucial?

When you work for your goals, your mental fortitude might help you feel less afraid of failing. When you experience loss or encounter other difficult situations, it can also be helpful. It's how you handle particular problems, followed by how quickly and effectively you recover.

You can develop your mental fortitude over time. The secret is to practice self-care, create a loving inner dialogue, and establish healthy coping mechanisms.

Methods for enhancing mental toughness

1. Recognize your emotions

It's crucial to be able to check in with yourself and identify your emotions. Because you can't begin to start giving yourself more of what you might need without that mental check-in.

2. Put self-compassion into practice.

Try practicing self-compassion if you're scared you insulted an in-law or weren't as patient with your child as you intended to be.

The objective is to calm your inner critic and treat yourself with kindness and gentleness, just as you would treat a friend.

Practice speaking to yourself like you would someone you truly care about when they are having a problem—without being critical of yourself. And extend the same compassion and love to others.

3. Identify your challenge.

Facing a difficulty? Inhale deeply and consider whether this is actually a tragedy or just a minor annoyance.

Small moves in the direction of what you want to avoid

When you're worried or depressed, you usually try to stay away from activities you find unpleasant. You might also put something off. (Hello, presentation for work.)

However, work on taking baby steps toward the circumstance or task rather than completely avoiding it. Would you be able to set aside an hour every day for that presentation?

Not only will practicing taking modest steps assist to reduce anxiety, but it can also boost your attitude and self-confidence.

4. Practice being mindful.

It's a good idea to remember and practice mindfulness when you're stressed or feeling anxious. Give yourself room to breathe and consider your responses.

To stay present, try box breathing or a one-minute meditation.

Learn techniques that will enable you to be more present. It can be quite beneficial to learn how to breathe and to experience the present through your breath.

5. Externalize your emotions

Do not suppress your emotions if anything is bothering you. Work on communicating your feelings in an authoritative manner.

Having a supportive and empowering social network as well as the discipline of acknowledging your feelings and effectively articulating them, whether through journaling, counseling, or talking to your best friend, is very important.

6. Keep up a fit lifestyle

Exercise, a balanced diet, and getting enough sleep are all things you can do to live a healthy life. These things can also help you be more emotionally resilient.

Without maintaining a regular sleep schedule, I don't think it's possible to be mentally strong or emotionally resilient. Limit your use of social media and news sources as well.

10 Exercises to Develop Mental Toughness

1. Use a cold shower

Each expert we spoke to connected mental toughness to the capacity to put up with discomfort, whether it be psychological or bodily. A quick, though not straightforward, approach to become more accustomed to discomfort is to begin or end each day with a cold shower.

We improve our immune system's function, blood circulation, and endocrine function when we take cold showers. In the yogic tradition, the cold shower is a recommended element of one’s daily morning practice. It stimulates the neurological system, nourishes the capillaries, and develops mental tenacity.

It's challenging to enter a freezing shower. For those who are up for the task, however, it will not only serve as continual training in both physical and mental toughness, but it will also provide you an endorphin rush and extra energy for the day.

2. When you are hungry, wait a few minutes before eating.

Allowing oneself to experience hunger pangs without reaching for a snack is another easy technique to develop a tolerance for discomfort (and impulse control).

It develops patience to put up with an additional five to ten minutes of hunger. "You can accept that waiting and being hungry are OK since you know you will eat. But instead of jumping in to repair it, you choose to sit with it. Your tolerance for discomfort increases as a result. You'll be able to handle more demanding problems if you're able to do that.

3. Make the Decision You Don't Want to Make (for 10 Minutes)

Tell yourself you only have to do anything for 10 minutes when it's something you really don't want to do, like exercise or a tedious report. When the 10-minute mark comes, give yourself permission to stop if you want to. (You'll probably keep going; getting started is generally the hardest.)

Beginning a task you don't want to do teaches your brain that you don't have to act on your feelings. You can still do something even if you don't feel like doing it. You are more capable than you realize; you have the ability to act even when unmotivated.

This also holds true for accepting bigger difficulties. Accept the challenge whenever your mind attempts to persuade you out of doing anything (like giving a presentation or attempting a new pastime).

Your brain undervalues you, claims Morin. "However, each time you accomplish a task you previously believed you were incapable of, you put your brain to the test and force it to start viewing you as more capable and competent than it already does.

4. Exercise without any music or TV

Of course, exercising is a fantastic way to increase both your physical and mental power. However, if you're doing it while watching TV or listening to music, you're depriving yourself of the chance to experience discomfort and develop a tolerance for it. Turn off your phone or iPad and focus more on your breathing and physical sensations while being present with your suffering.

Your capacity to develop grit is maximized when you exercise while distracted. If you already exercise in a distraction-free environment, take it a step further by include a mantra in each repetition, step, or breathe. Some people find that using phrases like "Let go" or "Thank you" makes them feel more at ease.

5. Ponder Your Emotions

The next time you begin to feel alone, irate, angry, anxious, sad, afraid, or envious, take a moment to breathe. Take note if you were ready to turn on the Xbox, pick up a beer, or grab your phone to check your email or look through Instagram. Resist the impulse to stand up and instead sit or lie down (face down is preferable), then close your eyes. Find a physical sensation in your body if you can. Do you experience any chest discomfort? Inside of you? Your heart is beating fast? Do you have a sore throat? Do you have a tight jaw?

Whatever feeling you discover, give it your full attention. Put aside the racing thoughts and refrain from attempting to identify your feelings if they are muddled. Simply immerse yourself in the sensation and give it your best. Spend some time with the bodily sensation. Then inquire as to what it is attempting to convey.

Although it may sound strange, this technique is employed in both traditional yogic practices and somatic-based psychology. This will provide you a surprising amount of insight, and you'll probably stop yourself from engaging in your harmful habit of ignoring your emotions.

One of the hardest things we'll ever have to do is to sit with our feelings. Some people find it simpler to engage in conflict than to experience emotion. But the best results frequently come from the hardest tasks. And according to Arrington, this exercise will not only increase mental toughness but also enhance your relationships, assist in the healing of past traumas, help you kick badly habits, and advance you to the next stage of personal growth.

6. Name Your Feelings Right Now (and Throughout the Day)

It can be challenging to describe your sentiments in words. Even admitting to yourself that you are anxious or depressed may be difficult. But according to study, giving your feelings names makes them less painful. So set alarms on your phone for the morning, afternoon, and evening and check in with yourself a few times throughout the day to see how you're doing.

You'll feel better if you can identify the mood or combination of emotions. It might only include pausing for a moment and naming your feelings to yourself.

Write them down using a pen and paper or take notes on your phone. You can also use a list of words for emotions to help you describe your emotions. Connecting with your emotions is crucial if you want to understand how they influence your choices. When you're upset or embarrassed, you might take significant risks that are unnecessary.

7. Inhale deeply

Deep breathing is vital for enhancing mental toughness, whether it is done formally during meditation or on an as-needed basis. When things get tough, it enables you to better control your thoughts, feelings, and, well, breathing. You may relax by reducing the amounts of cortisol in your body and brain, which are impairing your ability to think clearly.

While deep, leisurely breathing calms you down and lowers your cortisol and adrenaline levels, hyperventilating can make you feel worse. It gets your stress response to work for you rather than against you, getting you ready to take effective action. There are two ways to breathe: the 10-second pause, which involves taking three deep breaths and exhaling them after holding your breath for seven seconds; and the box breathing technique, which involves taking four deep breaths and holding them for four seconds before exhaling them after holding them for four seconds. You can also breathe in one nostril and out the other. "The oxygen flow from deep breathing aids in resetting the biochemistry and innermost areas of your brain.

8. Speak with someone

Being a strong person versus appearing tough are two very different things. Pretending you have no troubles is part of acting strong. Admitting you don't have all the answers is a sign of strength. Even though it could be awkward, talking to someone might make you stronger and more resilient.

So, make an effort to connect with and communicate with your friends and family frequently. A close friend or relative may be able to provide you a different viewpoint on what you're going through. But be receptive to expert assistance. Get a referral to a mental health expert after speaking with your doctor to rule out any physical health issues. A therapist can now be reached via text, video chat, or phone.

9. Possess gratitude

According to studies, being appreciative has a variety of advantages, including an increase in immunity, better sleep, and greater mental fortitude. You can strengthen your mind by seeking out something each day for which to feel grateful. Make it a habit to reflect on the things you are grateful for, either before you get out of bed in the morning or before you go to sleep. Finding the bright side influences our worldview and is a key component of developing mental toughness.

10. Admit Your Errors

When they know they've done something wrong, people typically try to deny their faults even happened, but mentally tough people never do this. Many people try (futilely) to defend their position rather than simply recognizing their mistake. This merely widens the gap, destroys connections, and causes trust to be lost. People with strong mental faculties take full responsibility for their acts rather than being too proud to admit they were mistaken. Acknowledging your errors releases you from guilt.

Acknowledging errors also sets a positive example for your children. When we make mistakes in front of our kids as parents, we frequently feel bad about it. However, we shouldn't strive to hide our mistakes or let our guilt and shame to rule us. Instead, we should reframe our failures as useful learning experiences that will better equip our kids to successfully negotiate the challenging aspects of life. We must have the courage to own up to our mistakes and the fortitude to correct them and move on. We must instill in our kids the importance of being open, honest, and vulnerable as well as how to use failure as a springboard for improvement.

Conclusion
The importance of mental health

Mental wellness is important. Maintaining good mental health helps us be resilient and bounce back from any setbacks.

A bad day can happen to everyone, but it doesn't necessarily indicate a horrible life. What matters is how we handle it and take care of our mental health.

www.ingramcontent.com/pod-product-compliance
Lightning Source LLC
LaVergne TN
LVHW052108160826
845678LV00015B/3431

* 9 7 9 8 3 5 2 1 1 4 2 5 4 *